# Mail Order Form

## — Workstation Radiation —

Additional copies of this book are available from:
Weldon Publishing
P.O. Box 4146
Prescott, AZ 86302

Price:      $7.95 plus $1.50 shipping charge
per book.

Sales Tax:  Arizona residents, please add
40 cents per book.

Ship to:

Name: _____

Address:_____

City:_____State: _____

Zip Code: _____

Please enclose check or money order payable to
Weldon Publishing.

# WORKSTATION RADIATION

*How to Reduce
Electromagnetic Radiation
Exposure from Computers,
TV Sets, and Other Sources*

Lucinda Grant

Weldon Publishing
Post Office Box 4146
Prescott, AZ 86302


ISBN 0-9635407-1-8

Library of Congress Catalog Card Number: 92-85285

Printed in the United States of America

First Edition

*One who is fighting most* *

to regain health

knows most the value of it.

*In memory of my mother,*

*Marjorie W. Grant,*

*whose love will always*

*be a beacon of hope.*

## About the Author

Lucinda Grant was graduated magna cum laude from Arizona State University with a BS degree in finance. She currently holds professional designations in financial planning and real estate.

Her investigation into electromagnetic radiation emissions began after she developed a chronic skin condition that intensified near computer monitors and TV sets.

Information obtained through her investigation that may be beneficial to others is what this book is about.

# Table of Contents

## *Terminology*

*The word "computer" as used throughout this book means the computer monitor, video display terminal (VDT), or computer display - specifically meaning the television-like display component of a computer system.*

*Glare screens, in general, mean computer display screen attachments which diminish screen glare but do not necessarily block radiation. Glare screens with electromagnetic reduction features, also known as anti-radiation screens, are the type specifically referred to throughout this book.*

## Product/Liability Disclaimer

This book represents knowledge the author or others have found to be valuable, or from resources believed to be reliable. However, the author is not an engineer, doctor, or scientist.

Everyone is different and electronics vary. Therefore, the product information, office arrangements, etc. presented within this book may not necessarily be most beneficial for you. For your protection, seek a respected computer room engineer, technician, and/or other appropriate persons to guide you in determining how to best handle your computer arrangements, attachments, compatibility issues, etc.

Also, investigate warranties and refund policies prior to purchasing any products, for your further protection. The products mentioned herein are examples of what is available, but is by no means an exhaustive list. Check with your computer supplier for what may be obtained locally and for comparison purposes.

No advertising fees were accepted from businesses mentioned and no endorsement or recommendations of products or businesses is intended. Their product claims are strictly their own.

The author and the publisher are not responsible for any damage or loss of any kind occurring from information in this book, including errors and omissions. The information contained herein is only meant to suggest possibilities and cause the reader to seek proper reliable advice as pertains to his/her individual situation.

# Introduction

With the proliferation of computers in our world today, we need to be aware of our indoor environment to minimize exposure to an invisible environmental pollution: low-level electromagnetic radiation.

The controversial issue of whether these computer emissions are in any way harmful to computer users has produced strong advocates on both sides with the general public caught in the middle – wondering who to believe while using the very same computers in question. And, should we only wonder about the computer user? How far away from computer displays must a worker be in order to avoid such radiation?

Now is the time for examining your computer practices and implementing preventative measures to reduce unnecessary radiation exposures. Because computer radiation is not the only way we receive electromagnetic doses, methods to reduce exposure from other office and home sources are also included in this book.

# Chapter One

# Reducing Computer Emissions at the Source

Remember when your mother told you not to sit too close to the TV set? Well, maybe she was right after all! The technology of television sets is similar to most computer displays. Both can produce various kinds of electromagnetic radiation including ultraviolet, microwaves, soft x-rays, radio waves, infrared, visible light, low frequency electrical and magnetic fields.[14 24 26]

Most types of actual computer and TV set emissions are considered very low. For instance, the ultraviolet exposure from computers is often much less than from fluorescent lights. The computer monitor's casing reduces the soft x-rays; if any soft x-rays are emitted they usually would be weak and not generally considered a health risk. Computer and TV set emissions meet current U.S. radiation regulations or guidelines unless the unit is damaged, defective, or an older model (before 1970 laws). However, recent concern has centered on the possibility of the low frequency electrical and magnetic fields creating adverse health effects.

Note: Numbered references throughout the text indicate sources for further study. (See Bibliography, page 91.)

Some people have reported experiencing various health disorders that they claim are aggravated by being near computer monitors (and sometimes TV sets, too): eye pain, skin rashes, nausea, headaches and fatigue. Some of the more serious health-related problems also questionably linked to computer use include cataracts, miscarriages, and cancer.[4][6][11][14] Whether these health problems are in any way caused or promoted by any computer radiation emissions is an ongoing debate.

Reports of possible computer-related health problems have occurred in the U.S., England, Canada, Sweden, and other countries. Over one hundred computer users in the Scandinavian countries acquired an acute skin rash that intensified near computers. Static electricity fields at the monitor were suspected of contributing to the skin rashes.[14][26] These rashes, which usually appear on unclothed areas of the skin – face, hands, arms – may be affecting very light-skinned people more. Their skin normally would be more sensitive to ultraviolet radiation (sunlight) than darker-skinned people. Although ultraviolet is not necessarily a contributing factor in this case, skin pigment variations may play a determining factor in the skin's sensitivity to the environment.

In part because of the skin rash problem, Sweden has the world's most restrictive computer standards, particularly in the monitor's low frequency electrical and magnetic field emissions.[19][26] In Sweden, special emphasis has been placed on reducing the extremely low frequency (ELF) and very low frequency (VLF) electrical and magnetic fields, as well as reducing static electricity. Some U.S. computer monitors meet Sweden's stricter standards, but many do not, especially older computers now in wide use.

Apple (1-800-776-2333), IBM (1-800-772-2227), and Safe Technologies Corporation (1-800-638-9121) are among those that claim to be marketing some lower-radiation monitors with reduced low frequency electrical and/or magnetic fields.

Check with your local computer supplier or the manufacturer to determine whether your particular monitor has modifications to meet <u>Sweden's MPR2</u> electrical and magnetic field reductions. Specifically ask whether these fields meet the current Swedish emission guidelines:

- Static electricity

- Extremely low frequency (ELF) electrical field

- Extremely low frequency (ELF) magnetic field

- Very low frequency (VLF) electrical field

- Very low frequency (VLF) magnetic field

The Swedish magnetic field reduction guidelines use a series of measurements around the front, back, and sides of the monitor to determine compliance. You may find that your monitor's magnetic fields are reduced, but not the electrical ones. Unless a grounded conductive coating has been applied to the screen, electrical fields can emanate freely from the front of the monitor, even if internal electrical shielding reduces the back/side areas. A glare screen with electrical reduction features can lessen low frequency electrical fields at the front of the monitor and static electricity.

Electromagnetic emissions still occur in monitors meeting the Swedish standards, but the fields the Swedish considered most potentially potent have been reduced. Whether these or other fields have been diminished enough or need to be diminished at all has not been scientifically proven.

The wide computer display box that looks like a TV set is generally a cathode-ray tube (CRT) monitor. They produce the same types of electromagnetic radiation as TV sets.

The slim display boxes of liquid crystal displays (LCD) do not use technology that produces x-rays, but can emit low frequency electrical and magnetic radiation. LCDs are usually small laptop computers. Laptops may also be gas plasma displays, which emit electrical/magnetic fields too.

Shielding attachments, such as glare screens, are not commonly available for laptops but the Swedish guidelines could still be checked out to determine your exposure. Reduce exposure to laptop computer emissions by not using them on your lap. Place them instead on a desk at a comfortable reading and typing distance.

If you want to check ELF and VLF computer emissions for yourself, several meters are available for rental or purchase. Because scientific studies have focused on possible health effects of magnetic fields, particularly the ELF magnetic field, meters available mainly measure these fields. Ask to be sure your meter will include instructions for assessing Swedish standards for the meter's field measurements. A meter may also be useful when shopping for your next computer display or for testing office arrangements discussed in the next chapter. ELF magnetic field meters can measure power line and appliance magnetic field emissions too. VLF magnetic field meters are used to measure these higher energy fields from computers and TV sets only. (See Sources, page 25.)

Once you find out whether your computer monitor meets the Swedish MPR2 radiation standards for these fields, you will know how to proceed in determining what shielding techniques are applicable in your case. Having a lower-radiation monitor helps minimize emissions at the source.

Computer shielding is primarily designed for CRT monitors. Multicolored CRT screens often produce more emissions than the usual monochromatic CRTs.

If your present monitor meets Swedish ELF and VLF radiation standards, you could consider further reducing the CRT's emissions at the screen. Some glare screens claim to reduce static electricity, soft x-rays, or ultraviolet emissions at the front of the monitor in addition to glare reduction. (See Sources, page 22.)

If your computer does not meet Sweden's standards, you may want to investigate various electrical and magnetic field alterations available for external or internal application. Computer shielding may involve a glare screen with electromagnetic reduction features for the front, with internal and/or external metal shielding for further reducing emissions.

First investigate whether your monitor's warranty will be affected, before having a computer technician apply internal shielding. Allow only a well-informed computer technician to make any internal alterations to your computer. Even if you unplug the monitor, stored voltage can be present so do not open the monitor casing yourself. You could be electrocuted or void the monitor's warranty.

ELF and VLF magnetic fields are particularly tricky to diminish. They easily penetrate office walls and practically everything else. Lead, which can block x-rays, can not stop these low frequency magnetic fields. Some computer manufac-turers are using a highly magnetizable metal composite, like Mu ( M•u ) metal, to help reduce magnetic field emissions. [3238] Mu metal is applied internally by the manufacturer, or by a highly trained computer technician later on. The internally applied Mu metal reduces emissions on all sides by attracting part of the magnetic field rather than blocking it. Glare screens cannot diminish magnetic field emissions in the ELF range; the screen would need to have Mu metal characteristics (nickel/iron alloy) to affect low frequency magnetic fields at all.

Electrical ELF and VLF fields are much easier to reduce. Glare screens with a conductive coating and a grounding wire can drain off static electricity and low frequency electrical fields at the front of the monitor. Conductive metal shielding (copper, etc.) with a grounding wire attached has been shown to reduce electrical fields at the back and sides. Metal shielding or glare screens used to decrease electrical fields should be grounded for safety and improved performance. Due to the electrical hazard involved in properly grounding metal shielding, allow only a computer technician to apply such shielding.

With other computer screen or shield attachments that do not require electrical expertise for application, follow the manufacturer's instructions and seek well-informed assistance if needed. The monitor needs ventilation to prevent overheating so be careful not to block off air passages at the back.

Rather than investigating various shielding techniques, purchasing a newer, lower-radiation monitor may be another option if your present monitor does not meet Swedish standards.

• End Note •

Consumers should ask questions of computer manufacturers that get beyond the easy "yes/no" about Swedish standards with regard to their monitors. Many computer salespeople and company representatives do not yet have the information about emissions and Sweden's MPR2 guidelines to help you make informed decisions. If not, ask them who you can call at the manufacturer's to find out specifics regarding their range of reductions and the extent of those reductions.

## Summary of Alternatives
## for Reducing Computer Monitor
## Radiation Exposure

1. Investigate whether your computer monitor's ELF, VLF, and static electricity emissions meet Sweden's radiation standards (MPR2). The electrical and magnetic ELF and VLF frequencies should be diminished if your computer meets those standards.

2. A) If your monitor does not meet Swedish standards, investigate various ELF and VLF electrical and magnetic field alterations available for external or internal application. (See Sources, page 22.)

   B) Whether your computer monitor meets Swedish standards or not, you could consider adding a glare screen with electromagnetic shielding features. (See Sources, page 22.)

3. After you have minimized the emission levels as much as possible, you could rearrange your work area and neighboring areas to further reduce your radiation exposure. (See Chapter Two.)

### Not all shielding will fit all monitors – ask first to be sure yours will.

— Static Electricity - Glare screens with static protection should be metal mesh or metalized plastic, with a grounding wire, for best long-term electrical conductivity. Nylon mesh screens with a carbon coating were found to lose their static protection over time, in Swedish studies.

— ELF and VLF Electric Fields - Same as for static electricity above for screen shielding. Reducing emissions from the back/side monitor area would require internal and/or external application of electrically conductive metal ( copper, etc.) properly grounded, and for safety should only be handled by a qualified computer technician due to the potential electrical shock hazard.

— ELF and VLF Magnetic Fields - Glare screens of any type do not reduce this ELF field. Reduction usually requires a highly qualified computer technician to apply Mu metal (nickel/iron alloy) internal shielding, although an external ELF magnetic field reducer is available. The VLF magnetic field is usually reduced by internal Mu metal application.

— Soft X-rays and Ultraviolet - CRT monitors and TV sets are the intended market for these shields. However, the Radiation Control for Heath and Safety Act of 1968 has already required manufacturers to reduce these emissions significantly. Color screens are more apt to produce these fields, although actual emissions are tightly regulated at the point of manufacture. TV sets and CRTs manufactured prior to the effective date of these laws (before 1970) are the most suitable candidates for such shielding.

Scientific Note:

ELF magnetic field emissions are limited to 2.5 milligauss (mG) and the VLF magnetic field limited to .25 milligauss (mG) under the Swedish standards, both measured at 20 inches from the display. These limits are mentioned here only for comparing to what extent lower-radiation monitors meet these guidelines, when discussing the limits with monitor manufacturers. Before measuring these yourself, specifically ask your meter's manufacturer how to measure the Swedish standards with your meter, as the calculation for these limits varies depending on your meter's sophistication.

The Swedish Confederation of Professional Employees labor union and the New York City Board of Education school system require their monitors to meet ELF magnetic field standards even stricter than the Swedish standards: 2 milligauss at 12 inches from the computer screen. Levels below one milligauss are preferable.

### Sources
#### — Shielding —

— Fairfield Engineering
   3007 West Grimes
   Fairfield, Iowa 52556

   Phone:  1-515-472-5551
   Fax:     1-515-472-4359

- ELF magnetic field reducer for internal application-requires installation by a computer technician.

— Inmac
2465 Augustine Drive
P.O. Box 58031
Santa Clara, CA 95052

Phone:  1-800-547-5444
        1-214-647-8298 (Dallas)
Fax:    1-214-641-1874 (Dallas)

- Glare screen with x-ray shielding,
  ELF and VLF electric shielding,
  and static protection.


— I-Protect, Incorporated
6151 West Century Blvd., Suite 916
Los Angeles, CA 90045

Phone:  1-800-733-2537
        1-213-215-1664
Fax:    1-213-215-9204

- Glare screen with x-ray and ultraviolet shielding.

— No-Rad Corporation
1549 11th St.
Santa Monica, CA 90401

Phone:  1-800-262-3260
        1-310-395-0800
Fax:    1-310-458-6397

- Glare screen with ELF/VLF electric shielding, static protection, microwave reduction, and other electric field shielding.
- External ELF magnetic field reducer.
- Glare screen (mesh) with ELF/VLF electric shielding, static protection, microwave reduction, partial higher frequency magnetic field shielding.

— Safe Technologies Corporation
145 Rosemary St.
Needham, MA 02194

Phone:  1-800-638-9121
        1-617-444-7778
Fax:    1-617-444-9528

- Internal shielding application to reduce ELF and VLF magnetic fields.
- Glare screen with ELF/VLF electric shielding and static protection.
- Product line includes pre-shielded, lower-radiation CRTs and an LCD monitor claimed to be fully blocked.

— Meters —

— Klabin Marketing
115 Central Park West
New York, NY 10023

Phone:   1-800-933-9440
         1-212-877-3632

- ELF meter for electrical and magnetic field measurements, with microwave setting.

— No-Rad Corporation
1549 11th St.
Santa Monica, CA 90401

Phone:   1-800-262-3260
         1-310-395-0800
Fax:     1-310-458-6397

- ELF magnetic field meter, and electrical field meter.

— Safe Technologies Corporation
  145 Rosemary St.
  Needham, MA 02194

  Phone:   1-800-638-9121
           1-617-444-7778
  Fax:     1-617-444-9528

  • ELF and VLF meters for magnetic field measure-
    ments.

Meters vary in price and range of sensitivity.The preced-
ing meters listed are among the least expensive (under
$200), and are intended for approximate measurements by
non-scientists.

More sophisticated, more expensive ELF meters are also
available, for institutional use, scientific experimentation, etc.
These are obtainable from various scientific instrument companies, such as the following:

— Davis Instrument Manufacturing Co.
  4701 Mount Hope Dr.
  Baltimore, MD  21215

  Phone:   1-800-368-2516
           1-410-243-4301

# Chapter Two

# Office Arrangements to Reduce Computer Radiation Exposure

After the source – the computer monitor – is minimized in emissions, further reduction of exposure levels can be obtained by office rearrangement.

These office arrangements may be particularly important because magnetic field energy is difficult to reduce. Distance from the source of magnetic fields is the best defense. [6] [11] [26] [28] Increasing space around computer workstations can reduce other radiation exposures, not just low frequency magnetic fields. The following office arrangements may be especially important if the office computer monitors do not meet Sweden's radiation emission standards.

### Office Arrangements:

If you are able to start an office policy regarding computer workstation arrangements, it may help initiate the office changes and keep those arrangements in place for everyone's benefit.

1. Turn off both the computer display and the disk drive box (or CPU-central processing unit) when you are not using the computer. This method should produce the same effect as unplugging them – eliminate the radiation by controlling the source.

Many office workers leave their monitors on all day at their desk whether the computers are being used or not. Presumably, this practice is for convenience. However, if your work requires intervals of computer work and computer inactivity, turning off the inactive equipment can diminish radiation exposure.

This method will conserve electricity as another benefit. The nationwide electrical requirements of powering computer monitors is huge, whether the machines are actively in use or not. In response to government urging, several computer manufacturers are designing monitors with a power reducer, activated automatically when the monitor is not being used. These more energy-efficient models will be out shortly.

By turning off the monitor and disk drive box instead, you are one step ahead of this technology.

2. Another radiation reduction option is to isolate the computer area from other tasks rather than having monitors dispersed throughout the offices. On the other hand, computer rooms can impose secondary radiation exposure possibilities if several computer displays are involved and spacing is not adequate. (See Arrangement Diagram #4, page 40.)

When you turn off your monitor/disk drive box or transfer

them to a lesser used area of the building, you may notice that you stay cooler while away from them as computers elevate the room temperature while on. You may also feel less stressful because your body will have less indoor environmental pollution to deal with.

3. Next, you could consider how to arrange your desktop computer system so that you are comfortable and have maximized your distance from it. To do so, place the computer monitor as far away as you can comfortably read it. Computer software that enlarges letter size (Eye Relief, etc.) and attachable keyboard drawers help to increase that distance.

Because the disk drive box also emits magnetic radiation when on, place it as far away from you as possible. Use an extension cord, if you can. Be sure the extension cord meets your computer's electrical requirements and complies with local fire code regulations. Check with your computer supplier.

The disk drive box is often situated directly under the computer's display screen at the person's desk. This is unnecessary and only subjects you to additional magnetic field radiation. Stands are available to hold the disk drive box on the floor away from you.

When you remove the disk drive box from underneath your monitor, the screen may be too low for your comfort. Adjustable arm attachments can elevate the computer display over your desk to add space. Also, elevating the monitor to eye level is one method recommended by ergonomic experts for reducing neck/back strain problems. Ergonomics means comfortably accommodating the workplace to the individual worker's needs.

Ergonomic design of each workstation is an important consideration that may eliminate health problems later on. Check with an ergonomic specialist if your workstation area cannot be comfortably arranged. They will advice you regarding chair type, chair position, monitor and keyboard height, and other workstation adjustments that can reduce your stress and strain. Wrist rests are an inexpensive, comfort necessity for a well designed workstation to help prevent the repetitive-motion injury, carpal tunnel syndrome. Wrist rests position the wrists straight at the computer keyboard. (Check with your computer supplier or see Sources, page 32.)

4. Another office pattern that is widespread involves placing CRT computer monitors back-to-back. Magnetic fields can be measured behind and beside computers as well as in front of them. Magnetic field emissions behind the monitor are stronger than at the front due to the position of the flyback transformer.

To reduce your magnetic field exposure from monitors other than yours, space yourself as far away from other computers as you can. Doing so will reduce the multiple exposures possible when sitting close to several computers operating at once. For example, a non-profit organization called Fund for the City of New York arranged their computer users about 28 inches from their screens and about 40 inches from other computer monitors. [6] [14] Municipal employees for the City of New York used union contract negotiations to get similar workplace standards.

Because emissions generally exceed those distances, Safe

Technologies Corporation, a computer shielding company, has recommended computer users distance themselves at least seven feet from other displays to diminish secondary radiation exposure. If space allows, stretch out for comfort and reduced exposures. (See Arrangement Diagrams #1 through #4, pages 34-41.)

In stockbroker and travel agency offices particularly, monitors are often placed with the back or side very close to the visiting customer. To reduce your customers' electrical/magnetic field exposure, arrange your monitor and their chair so that a comfortable distance exists between the two, and the back/side computer area is vacant. (See Arrangement Diagram #5, page 42.)

## Sources

— Computer Accessories —

— Inmac
2465 Augustine Drive
P.O. Box 58031
Santa Clara, CA 95052

Phone:   1-800-547-5444
               1-214-647-8298 (Dallas)
Fax:       1-214-641-1874 (Dallas)

- Wide range of computer accessories including extension
  cords, monitor arms, disk drive box (CPU) stands, wrist
  rests, etc.

BETTER

OFFICE

ARRANGEMENTS

— Diagram #1 —

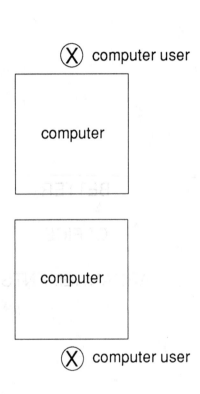

Usual Arrangement

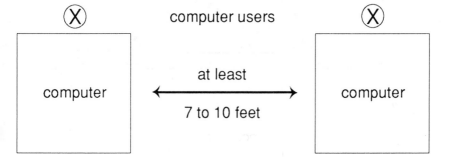

Better Arrangement

— Diagram #2 —

(X)  computer user

```
┌─────────────────┐
│                 │
│   computer      │
│                 │
│                 │
└─────────────────┘
```
                                    wall
═══════════════════════════════════════

```
┌─────────────────┐
│                 │
│   computer      │
│                 │
│                 │
└─────────────────┘
```

(X)  computer user

Usual Arrangement

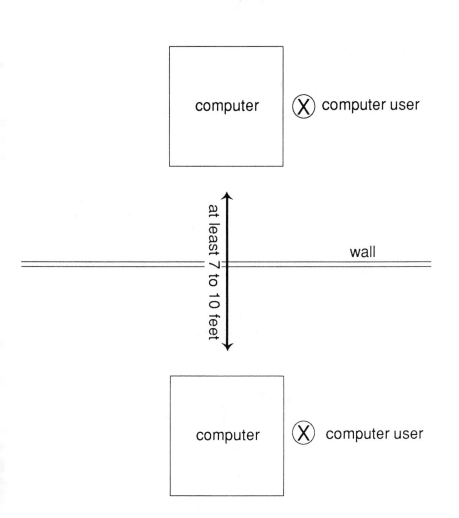

Better Arrangement

— Diagram #3 —

person sitting in
potential magnetic
(X)  ←  field
wall

computer

(X) computer user

Usual Arrangement

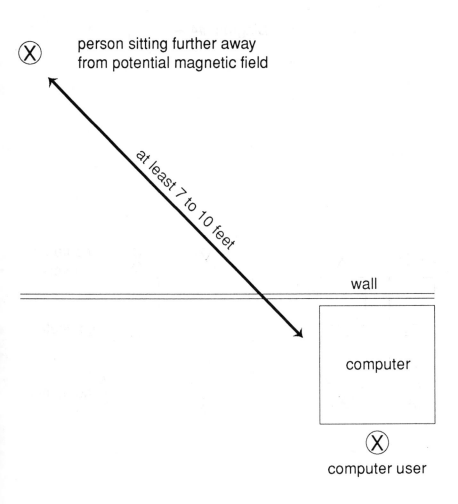

(X) person sitting further away
from potential magnetic field

at least 7 to 10 feet

wall

computer

(X)
computer user

Better Arrangement

— Diagram #4 —

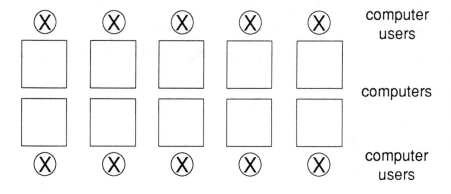

computer users

computers

computer users

Usual Arrangement

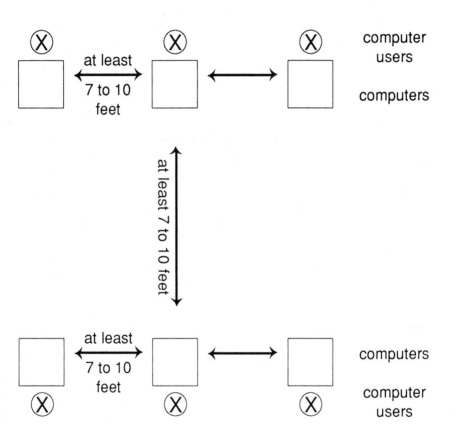

Better Arrangement

— Diagram #5 —

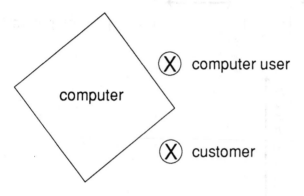

Usual Arrangement

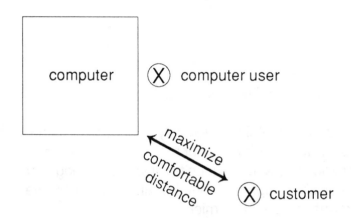

Better Arrangement

• End Note •

Mu metal means a metal that is highly permeable to magnetic fields; it provides an easy path for magnetic fields to travel
in.  It is often expensive and requires technical knowledge for
proper computer shielding.  Mu metal is also known by the
trademarks Permalloy and Hypernick.

# Chapter Three

# Home Arrangements to Reduce TV Set Radiation Exposure

As you reorganize your work environment to maximize your health, you will start to be more aware of what is around you, both at work and at home.

Because TV sets and CRT computers have similar technology and similar radiation emissions, you will want to check how the TV set relates to your home seating arrangements and rooms.

Preferably, the TV set should be backed against an outside wall because the electronics produce a stronger magnetic discharge out the back of the machine, like CRTs. To reduce radiation exposure, do not put a TV set against an inside wall where someone sits or sleeps directly behind that wall while the TV set is being used.

Newer TV sets that are turned off produce a lesser, but constant, electric and magnetic field force in order to interact with the remote control's infrared beam. If you have this type of TV set plugged in all of the time, avoid being directly behind it whether the TV set is actively being used or not in order to minimize unnecessary exposure.

If you sit off-center from the front of the TV screen, your exposure to the radiation activating the picture may possibly be reduced – especially with older, pre-1970 TV sets. [6] [11] (Sitting off-center from your CRT monitor may diminish exposure to the computer screen's radiation somewhat. However, this positioning can be uncomfortable due to the close distance involved and, therefore, is not ergonomically correct.)

Regarding the distance to sit from the TV set, radiation emissions generally reduce considerably at 10 feet. As long as you can comfortably see the TV's picture 10 feet away, you could sit at that distance to reduce exposure from TV radiation emissions. Children should not be allowed to sit up close to the TV set for the same reason. (See Arrangement Diagrams #6 and #7, pages 48 - 51).

BETTER

HOME

ARRANGEMENTS

— Diagram #6 —

TV set

(X) TV watcher

Usual Arrangement

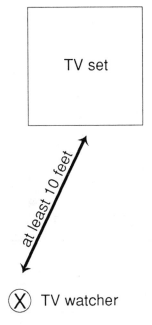

Better Arrangement

— Diagram #7 —

Usual Arrangement

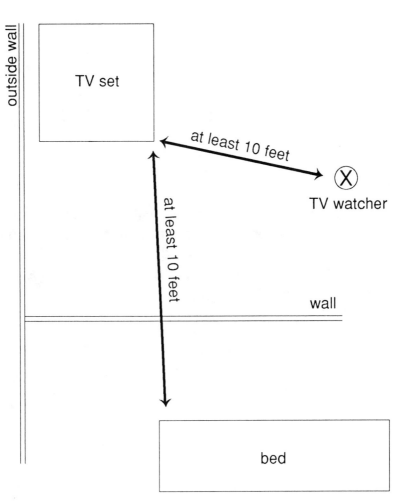

Better Arrangement

• End Note •

Large-screen LCD TV sets are in the developmental stages in Japan. However, problems with internal dust accumulation interfering with the electronics and picture clarity problems have slowed their progress. Tiny, portable LCD TVs are already available in the U.S.

# Chapter Four

# Additional Options Available to Reduce Radiation Exposure

Our modern world is continually being bombarded by new electronic gadgets. Some of the latest ideas include computer-assisted grocery carts and intra-office computer networking by radio waves. Needless to say, our daily electromagnetic dose will increase with such technology. Although each electronic product must meet whatever U.S. emission regulations apply to the technology, we are receiving overlapping doses from many sources.

Until scientists can determine specifically whether lower frequency radiation is harmful, minimizing your health risks could reduce your concerns about it and benefit your health at the same time.

Besides using the safest products you can find and afford, what do you do? Moving to a deserted island, of course, solves the radiation issue as much as it can be solved in today's world. (Satellite technology will even find you there.)

Man-made radiation takes many forms, several of which

you encounter daily: fluorescent lights, electric blankets, cellular phones, electrical power lines, electrical substations, and all electrical appliances to some extent, from the office copier to your refrigerator. Some of these items emit much lower electromagnetic radiation levels than others. Types of emissions may also vary. Plug-in appliances and electrical power lines emit ELF (extremely low frequency) electrical and magnetic fields. Wireless technology (radar guns, cellular phones, some home security systems, etc.) generally uses microwaves, radio waves, or sound waves.

What can you do to minimize this radiation exposure in the office and at home? The safest rule of radiation is avoidance. Stay away from unnecessary radiation sources as much as possible. Where these sources are under your control, you can decide whether to use them or substitute them for a more back-to-basics approach. For instance, using razors with razor blades instead of electric razors, regular toothbrushes and can openers instead of the electric variety are small ways to give your body a break from electrical/magnetic exposures.

Where avoidance is not possible, or inefficient/inconvenient, diminishment of your exposure to radiation sources is a good alternative.

You could consider ways to reduce your use of, or exposure to, daily electromagnetic sources such as the following:

**Electric Blankets**

If you unplug the electric blanket, you avoid prolonged unnecessary electrical and magnetic field exposure. Some studies of populations using electric blankets have shown a possible increased risk of breast cancer or miscarriage more than non-electric blanket users. * [6] [13]

Some manufacturers now make lower-radiation electric blankets with reduced magnetic field emissions. A better alternative is to wear socks, warmer nightclothes, and a warm sweatshirt to bed instead and add blankets. This method keeps you warmer when you get up and helps maintain body heat until the house warms up in the morning.

### Microwave Ovens

Try using a conventional oven, toaster oven, or stove instead of a microwave oven. This method minimizes irradiating your food and lessens magnetic field and microwave exposures.

If you do use a microwave oven at times, allow a distance of several feet between you and the operating oven.

### Appliances

To help your children reduce electromagnetic exposure, do not leave them near motorized appliances when the machines are in use. For example, keep cradles, playpens, baby seats spaced at a comfortable distance from the electrical refrigerator. For yourself, allow room to make meals at a table or counter that is not directly beside the refrigerator. The electric refrigerator's

* Electric Blankets and Breast Cancer: Report from the Society of Epidemiologic Research; Electric Blankets and Miscarriage: Nancy Wertheimer and Ed Leeper, University of Colorado at Boulder.

motor operates about one-half to three-quarters of the time. The emissions represent ELF electrical and magnetic field radiation; the magnetic field, in particular, is best avoided if possible.

## Outdoor Sources

Outside of the home, look for radio/TV tower transmitters, high-power electrical lines (metal poles), and electrical sub-stations. Distance yourself from these when locating a new place to live. If you already live near these electromagnetic sources, an ELF magnetic field meter can determine the extent of that field's exposure inside and outside the dwelling. [6] [28] Other emissions, such as radio waves and/or electrical fields, may also be present.

## Office Equipment

At work, to reduce your electromagnetic exposures further, do not place extra equipment on your desk. Arrange printers and fax machines away from your immediate work area. Because electric and electronic typewriters emit some ELF electric and magnetic field energy, turning them off when you are not using them avoids unnecessary exposure.

## Lighting

Office lighting is mostly of the fluorescent variety today. Fluorescent lighting emits various forms of electromagnetics, one of which is ultraviolet.

Some eye doctors are recommending contact lenses with

ultraviolet protection such as an outdoor variety, for computer users who have contact lenses. These lenses act like sunglasses, which block some ultraviolet exposure to the eyes. This ultraviolet protection may help reduce eye exposure to fluorescent lighting and computer screens. A computer glare screen that is specifically designed to shield ultraviolet rays may be useful for non-contact lens wearers. If you want to reduce the ultraviolet exposure of fluorescent lighting at the bulbs, at least two types of diffusing covers are available to block some of those rays. (Ask your lighting supplier or see Sources, page 61.)

Artificial light is less balanced than natural sunlight. Light rays representing ultraviolet and visible light (colors) are less evenly dispersed with artificial light than natural light. Sunglasses, glare screens, and fluorescent light diffusers can further unbalance artificial light. [21] [24]

In the book *Health and Light*, pioneer time-lapse photographer John Nash Ott described cell and plant sensitivity to certain artificial light exposures. [21] He demonstrated that plants need a natural light spectrum, like the sun, in order to grow and reproduce optimally. If certain light rays were not present in a plant's environment, the plant often would not fully develop.

Some scientists believe that we also are sensitive to quality of light as a biological stimulant. People with depression problems from inadequate sunlight in winter have used full-spectrum lighting to improve their mood. In Finland, where winter months are dark, full-spectrum lighting provides a more natural, balanced lighting in place of conventional indoor lights. (See Sources, page 61.)

Mild indirect stimulation of the eyes by natural light or similar lighting on occasion may be beneficial to health. Artificial light, from computer monitors, TV sets, and fluorescent bulbs enter our eyes also, often for several hours at a time. Whether this unbalanced artificial lighting is unhealthy for us has not been adequately studied.

## Clothing

Wearing nylon and other synthetic fibers draws static electricity to the body. [10] To reduce static build-up near computers, use natural cloth fabrics, such as cotton and wool, which are more electrically neutral. Women who wear nylons could replace them with cotton or wool blend tights to diminish nylon use at the monitor. (See Sources, page 62.)

A glare screen with static reduction features will further lessen your static accumulation, as will good room ventilation and higher humidity levels.

Antistatic floor mats with a grounding cord can discharge your body's static build-up near computers. When you step on these mats, your excess charge is drained away. However, wearing rubber-soled shoes prevents being grounded to the mat because rubber does not transmit electricity. A grounded antistatic table mat to touch at the monitor instead, or non-rubber soles used with the floor mat will help you discharge static electricity. These antistatic mats are made to safeguard the computer from your accumulated static charge which can inactivate it. These mats could be helpful for you as well.

**Jewelry**

Another way to reduce the possibility of accumulating electrical energy is to minimize wearing metal jewelry near computers. [11] [16] Wearing a metal necklace or metal bracelet at the monitor may cause the body to use the metal as an antenna to draw such energy to the body.

To help release excess electrical energy stored by the body, find time to walk barefoot on the bare ground or grass. [10] (In colder weather, dress warmly and sit or lie down on the ground instead.) This method will help ground the body's electrical system to the earth's natural low-level negatively charged electromagnetic field. (Conversely, computers and TV sets create a positively charged field.) According to the Environmental Health Center, a medical clinic for the electrically and chemically sensitive in Dallas, Texas (1-214-368-4132), extremely electrically sensitive people use this earth-grounding method during their recovery process.

Electrical sensitivity is not peculiar to man-made electronics. There are places throughout the world where seasonal winds, by friction, produce a high positive-charge static electricity field. The Sirocco in Italy and the Chinook winds in Montana are examples of this electrical disturbance. During these winds, residents tend to become more irritable and stressful. [10] [15] [23] [29]

One biological explanation for this increased irritability, as determined by studies in California and Israel, is that highly positively charged air can cause increased stress and addi -

tional serotonin production.* Serotonin is a neurotransmitter –
a chemical that transmits nerve impulses in the body's nervous
system.

According to these studies, when the body produces too
much serotonin, medical problems including eye irritation,
headache, nausea, dizziness, and sinus problems may occur
in some sensitive individuals. Interestingly some of these
complaints resemble those of computer users. The positively
charged indoor environment of our computer rooms could be a
factor in making some of us more stressful because of the
electrical imbalance present. [10] [14] [29]

Negative ion generators have sometimes been proposed as
one way to correct an excessive positive-charge indoor environment. However, these air cleaners/air rechargers can
sometimes emit small amounts of ozone, which is unhealthy in
larger quantities – caution is advised. [10] [28]

### • End Note •

The positive air ions of static electricity generated by computer monitors were suspected of initiating Sweden's skin rash
cases. Because opposite electrical charges attract, the positive ions attract to the computer operator's face and exposed
skin. Dust particles and airborne pollutants follow, which may
intensify skin reactions and eye irritations - particularly with
contact lens wearers. Glare screens with static protection were
the recommended solution in Sweden, but did not always
reverse the skin rash problem. [14]

* Albert P. Krueger, University of California at Berkeley; Felix G. Sulman, M.D., Hadassah
Medical Center, Jerusalem, Israel.

## Sources

— Lighting Components —

— Hart Lighting & Supply
3801 E. Roeser Rd., Suite 10
Phoenix, AZ 85040

Phone:   1-602-437-0375
Fax:      1-602-437-1264

• Two varieties of ultraviolet shielding for fluorescent
  lighting.

— L & H Vitamins, Inc.
37-10 Crescent St.
Long Island City, NY  11101

Phone:  1-800-221-1152

— N.E.E.D.S.
527 Charles Ave., 12-A
Syracuse, NY 13209

Phone:  1-800-634-1380

• Both companies above have full-spectrum light bulbs to
  install in incandescent fixtures.

— Natural Clothing Fibers —


— Garnet Hill
262 Main St.
Franconia, NH 03580

Phone:  1-800-622-6216

• Women's clothing – 100% cotton tights and several other tights in cotton or wool blends, instead of nylons.


— Lands' End, Inc.
1 Lands' End Lane
Dodgeville, WI 53595

Phone:  1-800-356-4444

• Women's clothing – 67% cotton blend tights, instead of nylons.

• Also men's and children's natural fiber clothing.

# Chapter Five

# Problems with Electromagnetic Radiation Studies

Electromagnetic radiation studies involving biological effects of low frequency fields have produced mixed results. Some studies seem to indicate potential health risks while others found no link between ELF or VLF electromagnetics and adverse health effects. Therefore, studies overall are called inconclusive.

Because of the highly technical nature of such studies, which include biology and physics, the general public cannot readily or reliably draw conclusions from any one individual study. A study's length of time, the radiation type and strength, the type of animal or cell being irradiated, and potential unknown contributing factors as lighting or environmental chemicals could all influence what results are obtained.

To what extent these animal and cell studies represent the human experience (computer users, etc.) is further in question regardless of the study results obtained.

A summary of basic scientific findings for some specific

computer field emissions follows:

## Ultraviolet

CRT computer displays generally emit less ultraviolet than fluorescent lights. According to the Lupus Foundation of America, Inc. (1-800-558-0121), lupus patients with sun sensitivity have not reported widespread computer-related skin reactions from computer emissions, but many do react to fluorescent lighting and older color television sets.

Although ultraviolet exposure may be very low for computer users, if you are looking into the screen for several hours at a time, a glare screen specifically designed to block some ultraviolet may help eye strain. (See Sources, page 22.)

## Microwaves

CRT computers do produce microwaves but the dose emitted is considered very small and almost unmeasurable. Microwave emissions at higher levels, from other sources, are being studied because of initial findings showing such possible biological effects as immune system suppression, cellular changes, and heart rate fluctuations. [6][14]

The former U.S.S.R. had a microwave emission exposure limit much smaller than the U.S. regulation in effect simultaneously. Maybe they know something we don't. For instance, Connecticut's State Police discontinued hand-held radar detectors, which emit microwaves, after some police officers claimed the radar detectors caused localized cancer. These officers believe that placing the radar gun near their body repeatedly over several years contributed to cancer developing at or near the radar gun's position.[22] No electromagnetic studies have been done yet concerning possible health effects from the radar guns in question.

Microwave testers to detect measurable leaks from your microwave oven can be purchased inexpensively at a local hardware store.

Microwave emissions from whatever source should be considered with caution, as some scientists believe exposure to radiation in general may be cumulative. Repeated exposures over long periods of time may reduce the body's ability to recover.

**Magnetic Fields**

Computer monitors (CRT, LCD, etc.) and TV sets can emit ELF (extremely low frequency) and VLF (very low frequency) magnetic fields. Sweden's computer emission standards limit both. Of these, the focus has largely involved biological effects possible from exposure to the ELF magnetic field. This field has been linked to promotion of cancer cell growth, immune system suppression, and nervous system problems, among others in biological studies.[6] [14] Electromagnetic studies have looked at occupations where electrical/magnetic field exposures are much higher than normal. Several of these studies show electricians and telephone linemen more at risk of brain cancer and leukemia than the normal population.[6] [14]

Also, scientific studies were made concerning the possible

cause of leukemia in Denver's children.* Their living arrangements suggested that the cancer was more common where magnetic field levels from electrical power line emissions were highest.[6][26]

Children may be more susceptible to electromagnetic exposures considering their size and more rapid cell growth than adults. Children are exposed to computer emissions at schools throughout the country. Hopefully, the computer emissions considered acceptable for adults will prove to be acceptable for children also. Otherwise, the long-term health implications could be very serious. As a precaution, their computer classrooms ideally would provide wide spacing between computer displays, lower-radiation monitors, and glare screens. (See Arrangement Diagram #4, page 40.)

Although magnetic fields are not necessarily a cause of cancer directly, some studies have shown that human colon cancer and breast cancer cells grew more easily than normal when magnetic fields were present. [6][14] Chemical pollutants in our air, water, and food may initiate the cell destruction to start this process.

According to a research report published by the National Cancer Institute, U.S. Department of Health and Human Services, colon cancer is the third most common cancer in the U.S. [18] Lung and skin cancer are more common. Their report states that the incidence of colon cancer tends to be proportionally more common in industrialized, heavily populated areas than

* Nancy Wertheimer and Ed Leeper, University of Colorado at Boulder; David Savitz, University of Colorado Medical Center.

in more remote locations. Perhaps pollution, both chemical and electromagnetic, are contributing factors.

Until we know for sure, ELF and VLF magnetic field emissions should be avoided or diminished when possible, in case present emission levels are found to be unsatisfactory.

### *Low Frequency Electromagnetic Emission Levels*

The strength of home and office appliance emissions vary with types and styles.

Higher

    Electrical substations
    High-power electrical lines (metal poles)
    Computer displays
    TV sets

Lower

    Refrigerators
    Automobiles
    Phones
    Battery-operated LCD clocks and calculators

Pregnant women should avoid all of the higher level exposures, and electric blankets, if possible. Some animal studies have shown embryos to be more sensitive to magnetic fields than the adult animals were. * [3] [14]

People with cancer probably should also avoid the higher

* Embryo Studies: Kaiser Permanente Medical Care Program, Oakland, CA; Alexander Martin, University of Western Ontario, London, Ontario, Canada.

emissions in order to reduce the possibility of magnetic fields promoting the growth of cancer cells, as some studies indicate. * 6 14

The embryonic and cancer cell studies, etc. may not necessarily be using emission levels you would be exposed to but for precautionary measures, avoidance is the best defense.


• End Note •


Our modern electrical power lines and appliances use pulsing, alternating current (AC) electricity. Our bodies produce direct current (DC) electricity instead, that can be measured in bodily function, such as the brain. The electroencephalograph (EEG) measures the electric field; new technology called SQUIDs (superconducting quantum interference devices) can detect the brain's small magnetic field for therapeutic purposes.

Stronger, higher frequency artificial ELF magnetic fields are suspected of interfering with the much weaker electricity of the body. Magnetic fields can induce weak electrical fields in electrical conductors, the body being such a conductor. This process, called induction, is theorized by some to be one way such fields may affect body chemistry.


* Cancer Promotion Studies: Jerry L. Phillips, Cancer Therapy and Research Center, San Antonio, TX; Johns Hopkins University, Baltimore, MD.

# Chapter Six

# Maximizing Health

Staying healthy by practicing healthy habits will help strengthen your body's immunity to environmental pollutants in our modern world.

Radiation, particularly sunlight and x-ray exposure, can promote free radical activity in the body. [20] [27] Free radicals are unbalanced molecule fragments that occur in the body through normal breathing and digestive processes. However, scientists are discovering that an excess of free radicals in the body may impair immunity and cause cellular deterioration, a beginning step to heart disease, cancer, and other degenerative diseases.

Current nutritional information indicates that some vitamins and minerals classified as antioxidants diminish free radical activity and, in effect, help protect cells from premature aging. Popular antioxidants include Vitamin C (in oranges), Vitamin E (in soybean oil), and beta carotene (a form of Vitamin A in carrots and squash). [17] [25] [27]

The National Cancer Institute (1-800-4-CANCER) strongly

recommends a <u>low fat, high fiber diet that includes at least five fruit or vegetable servings daily</u> as a possible cancer preventative measure. Their public awareness campaign called "5 a Day – for Better Health!" advocates fruit and vegetable sources for fiber and natural antioxidant protection, particularly from Vitamins A and C. (Wash or peel fruits and vegetables to minimize your pesticide intake. Pesticide-free foods are preferable.) Raw, fresh fruits and vegetables used as snacks or salads also provide enzymes which assist digestion and boost the immune system.

Several studies show that people who eat more fruits and vegetables are healthier than those who eat very few of them. At least one insurance company has taken the possibility of cancer prevention seriously by conducting a five-year study to investigate whether cigarette smokers and asbestos workers can reduce their lung cancer risk by taking beta carotene. [5]

Health food stores carry a wide variety of vitamin/mineral supplements if you feel you need more than your diet provides. Of course, check with your doctor before starting any type of diet supplementation program to make sure it is a good program for you – especially if you have a medical problem.

Conventional medical practitioners, such as your family doctor, are primarily educated in current pharmaceutical drugs and surgical techniques. They tend to know less about preventative methods like vitamins. On the other hand, your veterinarian probably knows a lot about how to use a balanced vitamin/mineral diet to promote the health of your dog or cat. An animal's diet determines energy levels, shine of the hair, and proportional weight. So too, we humans.

Moderate exercise, as well as proper food intake, helps cleanse and normalize body functions. The Chinese have used Tai Chi (Ti • Che), Qi Gong (Che • Gong), and other breathing/ exercise routines for centuries to assist healing and relieve daily stress. [12] [30]

Ask your doctor about your exercise potential, then find a suitable exercise regimen that you are comfortable with based upon your present health and try it. You'll feel better! For example, walking barefoot in the grass to ground yourself and reduce electrical excesses provides exercise as well.


• End Note •


Vitamin supplements can be harmful in large quantities. Be careful not to exceed the recommended daily amount listed on the label unless prescribed by a doctor, or sufficiently researched yourself so that you are aware of the upper limits and potential toxicity.

## Natural Vitamin A and C Sources*

| | Vitamin A | Vitamin C |
|---|:---:|:---:|
| **Fruits:** | | |
| Apricots (3) | x | |
| Cantaloupe(1/2 cup) | x | x |
| Grapefruit (1/2) | | x |
| Kiwi Fruit | | x |
| Orange | | x |
| Strawberries (1/2 cup) | | x |
| **Vegetables: (1/2 cup cooked)** | | |
| Bok Choy | x | |
| Broccoli | | x |
| Brussels Sprouts | | x |
| Carrots | x | |
| Cauliflower | | x |
| Spinach | x | |
| Sweet Potato | x | |
| Winter Squash | x | |

*All of the above are sources of fiber and contain at least 50% of the U.S. Recommended Daily Allowances (RDA) for the vitamin(s) indicated.

Source: National Cancer Institute, NIH Publication No. 92-3248

# Chapter Seven

# Making the Future
# a Healthier Place

Health issues in general will become more important as people become more product-aware and use their awareness to make healthy buying decisions. Increased customer awareness of product safety can persuade manufacturers to produce products with fewer questionable factors (chemicals, radiation emissions, etc.). Demand for improved products will provide market opportunities for both sellers and buyers whether or not we know the long-term health implications of these chemicals or electromagnetic fields in the short-term. By re-thinking the old and updating products to truly be user friendly, businesses could improve their environmental image and perhaps benefit public health, too.

In the workplace, we also need a higher awareness. Our indoor environments should display a more humane work setting where people and their office arrangement needs take precedence over furniture and wiring configurations.

This technological age has attempted to make human the machinery of industry. They can interact with other machines and with us. By doing so, the pace of the work has sped up. Let us not now robotize ourselves to accommodate the machinery. For example, computer monitoring practices that use electronic surveillance to determine clerical workers' computer productivity are using quantitative measurements. Where customer contact is involved, the question should not be how many, so much as how well, customers are handled. Random sampling of work by people may best provide that answer.

In summary, many computer workstation issues concerning worker health need to be dealt with by employers individually: job rotation (for variety and computer breaks to rest wrists/eyes, etc.), office redesign (for minimizing radiation exposure and improving ergonomic comfort factors), and a flexible office policy (allowing pregnant workers the option of non-computer work and accommodating job alternatives for those with possible computer-related health problems).

Some health problems such as back or wrist strain and eye discomfort may indeed be solved by the improved ergonomics of chair design, wrist rests, or glare screens. However, that leaves other problems such as skin rash, nausea, and miscarriage still under suspicion.

Many factors could adversely affect workers at the workplace besides computer emissions and they will need to be sorted out. Office lighting creating glare, ultraviolet exposure, and an unbalanced light spectrum are typical examples. Electrical energy creating static electricity, and the increased positive-charge indoor environment are further items to isolate in solving the computer radiation question. Chemicals in the air from copy machine paper and ink, carpeting, electronics exhaust, plastics, etc. may also be contributing factors to some at-work illnesses. On-the-job stress from electronic monitoring, poor workstation design, etc. add to the hidden potential factors affecting worker health.

Needless to say, isolating any specific irritating/unhealthy sources and determining allowable limits will probably take years. Protecting yourself from unnecessary chemical and radiation exposure during this technological transition is a good way to deal with the unknown.

Protective radiation options include computer shielding, office redesign, reducing exposure to non-essential electromagnetic sources, not wearing certain apparel/jewelry items near computer monitors, stress reduction, moderate exercise, and eating more fruits and vegetables (particularly those containing antioxidants).

## Sources

### — Computer Newsletter —

— VDT News
P.O. Box 1799
Grand Central Station
New York, NY 10163

Phone: 1-212-517-2802

• Reports on current computer-related health and safety issues around the world. Recommended for personnel departments responsible for a large computer-based workforce.

## –Computer Radiation
## Information Resources

— The Labor Institute
853 Broadway, Room 2014
New York, NY 10003

Phone:  1-212-674-3322

— Labor Occupational Health Program
University of California
School of Public Health
2515 Channing Way
Berkeley, CA 94720

Phone:  1-510-642-5507
Fax:      1-510-643-5698

APPENDIX

## Radiation Reactive Skin Rashes

Karolinska Hospital in Stockholm, Sweden studied many of Sweden's computer users with skin rashes. They questioned whether the rashes represented rosacea (roz • a • shah) or some other type of skin condition. Rosacea is a skin disease that produces redness, generally over the face, sometimes with rash or pimple formation. [9] [14]

Sweden's skin rash patients had the following symptoms which intensified near computer monitors: localized pain, red skin, itching, pimply rash. Some also further reacted to sun exposure or other electrical appliances.

Rosacea is known to be aggravated by sunlight, temperature extremes, stress, and certain foods that increase the body's warmth (spicy, alcoholic, or hot foods).

Sweden's patients may be able to benefit from the knowledge of others with a different radiation reacting skin disease. Discoid lupus erythematosus is an autoimmune disease with localized skin inflammation, usually on the face. Discoid lupus patients often experience intensified skin inflammation when exposed to ultraviolet sources (i.e., the sun, fluorescent light, older television sets). [1] [31]

Some lupus patients use natural Vitamin E (in addition to sunblock) applied directly to the affected area for reduced reactions. Vitamin E applied on the skin rash of computer users may also reduce their reactions. Vitamin E is widely known as a skin vitamin, for topical or oral use. [25] Topically applied, it can help protect cells from free radical damage directly at the injured site. Natural Vitamin E capsules are available at health food stores. To try reducing reactions, cut open a few capsules and apply the oil directly to the injured site, liberally and often, as needed.

Sweden's rash patients have found discontinued computer use and sometimes reduced use of other electrical appliances most helpful for reducing skin flare-ups.

Long-term chronic skin inflammation from whatever source can sometimes cause cancer. Therefore, reducing or eliminating contact with the primary skin irritants is advisable. Simply eliminating the rash's burning sensation with pain relievers is not enough; the reaction would still be occurring although you could not feel it. Better to avoid the irritants to help your skin heal.

What caused some people to have not only a burning skin reaction near computers, but a visible rash also? One possibility is that previous skin damage from the sun or other factors may have predisposed these computer users to later develop the skin rash condition. A deep sunburn can damage skin cells – cells that may not completely repair. These damaged cells may have a different, incomplete method of dealing with heat, in general.

Heat generated by the computer monitor, that the skin would normally be able to diffuse, may not be so efficiently handled by damaged cells. The heat reaction in damaged cells might cause the localized inflammation and eventually a rash as that skin area attempted to cool the cells. This damaged cell scenario may or may not be what Sweden's rash patients have endured, but is possible.

However and whenever their skin was damaged, the result is sometimes a recurring, radiation reactive, sunburn-like rash. Once this rash develops, several factors can trigger reactions – ELF magnetic fields, ultraviolet, and possibly static electricity and other factors. [14] So far, no cure is known but avoiding the triggering factors may help the healing process.

Further help for rosacea-type skin disorders might be found by consulting a naturopathic physician schooled in the use of natural treatments, such as vitamin therapy and herbs. Some herbs are helpful for skin disorders–burdock root, for instance. Specific, technical information concerning various herbs is available through The Herb Research Foundation (1-303-449-2265). Because herbs are often powerful medicine they may interact adversely with synthetic drugs and should only be used with a doctor's approval.

## Pinpointing Health Problems

Beyond Sweden's skin rash issue which seemed to indicate a direct cause/effect relationship between computer emissions and health, other health problems possibly related to computer emissions are less well scientifically documented.

For example, having fatigue or nausea may occur regardless of where you are. Therefore, pinpointing such a cause as computer radiation could be difficult, especially for worker's compensation benefits.

If you often feel less well at work than when you are at home during weekends, vacations, and holidays, you may be reacting to an unhealthy work environment which can contain both chemical and radiation pollution.

If so, you could try using a similar computer in the library or at home long enough to determine whether you notice a return of symptoms outside your work environment. This procedure may give you a clue as to whether the computer monitor seems to be aggravating the health problem.

Also, airborne chemical exposures in our indoor environments are widespread, particularly formaldehyde (carpeting) and phenol (electronics), which have caused chemical sensitivity problems for some people.

If you do find that you are less well at work or around

computers, minimize irritating exposures and seek a doctor who will consider your situation and symptoms seriously – preferably one who specializes in environmental illnesses, if you suspect chemical or electrical sensitivity.

## Electromagnetic Spectrum
(A selected list of fields in order of frequency)

Ionizing Radiation:          Gamma Rays
(Higher Frequency)           Hard X-rays
                             Soft X-rays
                             Ultraviolet

Non-Ionizing Radiation:      Visible Light
(Lower Frequency)            Infrared
                             Microwaves
                             Radio Waves
                             VLF (very low frequency)
                             ELF (extremely low frequency)

Ordinary household appliances usually emit ELF electrical and magnetic fields. CRT computer monitors and TV sets can produce the range of emissions from ELF through soft x-rays.

## Bioelectromagnetics

This investigation into electromagnetics and health often turned up the close and delicate relationship between cellular health and a properly functioning electrical system within the body.

According to some doctors and scientists, disease is more likely when the body's electrical system is malfunctioning [4] [7] [16]. Some, perhaps improperly, have further speculated that by inducing an artificial electrical current at the injured or diseased site, normal body electricity, and therefore healing, could be resumed.

For example, under certain conditions low frequency magnetic fields are known to influence calcium, magnesium, and potassium movements within the body. Using this knowledge, various experimental devices have been designed to promote healing of broken bones with directly applied pulsed magnetic fields, with some success.

Unfortunately, cancer cell growth also benefits from similar low level magnetic fields. [4] Whether there will be health problems from this type of bone-growth stimulating device is unknown, but does point out the power electricity has in influencing bodily functions.

While our Western medical practices seek to treat the result of disease, traditional Chinese medicine seeks to find the source of disease - what organs are not in balance - and correct that imbalance. Traditional treatment methods include herbs, massage, or acupuncture.

The Chinese believe that acupuncture uses energy pathways called Qi (Che), not nerve pathways. Qi means vital energy, which they believe is enhanced by daily exercise, a vegetarian diet, adequate rest, and Tai Chi or Qi Gong exercises to center this energy. [12][30] Tai Chi involves soft, dance-like body movements that are related to the martial arts. Qi Gong is similar to Tai Chi, but includes relaxation and meditation with special attention to deep breathing techniques. These traditional Chinese practices seem to be reinforcing the body's normal electrical flow. [4]

A positive mental attitude may also play an important part in maintaining the body's electrical potential: joy producing strong, healthy energy; depression, a likely suppressor of electrical current and health.

Bioelectromagnetics - the science of biological
electromagnetics - is not new.

In the early 1900's, a Russian engineer named Georges Lakhovsky experimented with electromagnetics as a healing agent. [16] He considered the natural electromagnetics of the earth itself useful to promote healing. If cells retained their electrical equilibrium, he believed they could overcome the foreign, differently oscillating electrical currents of disease.

Lakhovsky demonstrated these ideas by placing an open, but overlapping, circular copper antenna around plants that had fatal tumors. According to his theory, the copper ring drew the earth's electromagnetic energy to the plant's cells and helped the plant's normal cells resonate at their natural frequency to completely heal the plants. (It seems appropriate here to say that while drawing on the earth's natural electromagnetics may be healthy, metal cannot differentiate between natural fields and the myriad artificial electromagnetics pulsing in our environments today. Metal can also attract this higher frequency energy, which is certainly of a questionable nature relative to health, as previously discussed.)

While Lakhovsky lived in Paris, France he further demonstrated the importance of cellular equilibrium with his Multiple Wave Oscillator. This invention included an electromagnetic transmitter and a resonator which generated a variety of frequencies that he claimed allowed every cell to find its correct frequency and resonate accordingly.

His most striking success seems to be when he treated skin cancer patients with the Oscillator at the Hospital St. Louis, Paris in 1931. Fifteen minute applications over a period of 1 to 6 months brought complete healing to these patients, leaving only a scar.

Lakhovsky's ideas seemed to have proved themselves, based upon his plant and human cancer successes. While he treated other, internal illnesses with mild success, externally apparent illness seemed more easily treatable with the Oscillator. Unfortunately, his Oscillator methodology probably died with him in 1942.

Current cancer research and electromagnetic study should take serious note of such unconventionality in order to leave no stones unturned in redefining the everchanging limits of medicine and science.

We may find the Multiple Wave Oscillator technology useful for healing many types of skin problems.

## A Selected Bibliography

Those marked with an asterisk represent works dealing with the computer monitor/TV set radiation controversy.

1. Aladjem, Henrietta. *Understanding Lupus: What It Is, How to Treat It, How to Cope with It.* New York: Charles Scribner's Sons, 1985.

2. Barnothy, M.F., ed. *Biological Effects of Magnetic Fields.* Vol. I. New York: Plenum Press, 1964.

3. Barnothy, M.F., ed. *Biological Effects of Magnetic Fields.* Vol. II. New York: Plenum Press, 1969.

* 4. Becker, Robert O. *Cross Currents: The Promise of Electromedicine, the Perils of Electropollution.* Los Angeles: J.P. Tarcher, 1990.

5. Blue Cross Blue Shield of Oregon. "Researchers Recruiting Smokers for Cancer Study." *Health News Digest,* Spring 1991.

* 6. Brodeur, Paul. *Currents of Death: Power Lines, Computer Terminals, and the Attempt to Cover Up Their Threat to Your Health.* New York: Simon and Schuster, 1989.

7. Crile, George W. *The Phenomena of Life: A Radio-Electric Interpretation.* New York: W.W. Norton, 1936.

* 8. Cunningham, Ann Marie. "Electromagnetic Fields: In Search of the Truth." *Popular Science,* Dec. 1991.

9. Curatek Pharmaceuticals. *Rosacea: A Conspicuous Condition ... A Treatable Condition.* Elk Grove Village, IL: Curatek Pharmaceuticals, 1991.

10. Donsbach, Kurt W. D.C. Ph.D. and Morton Walker D.P.M. *Negative Ions.* Rosarito Beach, Baja CA, Mexico: Wholistic Publications, 1981.

*11. Dumpé, Bert. *X-rayed Without Consent: Computer Health Hazards.* Arlington, VA: Ergotech Assoc., Inc., 1989.

12. Elsenberg, David with Thomas Lee Wright. *Encounters with Qi: Exploring Chinese Medicine.* New York: Norton, 1985.

13. Gott, Peter M.D. "Electric Blankets Related to Breast Cancer.", *Prescott Courier,* Prescott, AZ, 11 May 1992.

*14. Hughes, Marija Matich MLS MHA. *Computer Health Hazards.* Washington, D.C.: Hughes Press, 1990.

15. Kals, W.S. *Your Health, Your Moods, and the Weather.* Garden City, NY: Doubleday, 1982.

16. Lakhovsky, Georges. *The Secret of Life.* Trans. Mark Clement. n.p.: True Health Publishing Co., 1951.

17. Murray, Frank. "Antioxidants: Health Allies." *Better Nutrition for Today's Living,* Oct. 1992.

18. National Cancer Institute. *Cancer of the Colon and Rectum Research Report.* Bethesda, MD: U.S. Dept. of Health and Human Services, March 1988.

*19. No-Rad Corporation Information Packet. Santa Monica, CA, 1992.

20. Nutrition News. *The Healthy Edge.* Pomona, CA: Nutrition News, 1986.

*21. Ott, John N. *Health and Light.* Old Greenwich, Conn.: The Devin-Adair Co., 1973.

22. Pane, Lisa Marie. "Connecticut First State to Ban Handheld Radar Guns." *Prescott Courier,* Prescott, AZ, 5 June 1992.

23. Persinger, Michael A., ed. *ELF and VLF Electromagnetic Field Effects.* New York: Plenum Press, 1974.

*24. Poch, David I. *Radiation Alert: A Consumer's Guide to Radiation.* Garden City, NY: Doubleday, 1985.

25. Prevention Magazine. *The Complete Book of Vitamins.* Emmaus, PA: Rodale Press, 1984.

*26. Safe Technologies Corporation Information Packet. Needham, MA, 1992.

*27. Schechter, Steven R. with Tom Monte. *Fighting Radiation with Food, Herbs, and Vitamins: Documented Natural Remedies that Protect You from Radiation, X-rays, and Chemical Pollutants.* Brookline, MA: East West Health Books, 1988.

*28. Smith, Cyril W. and Simon Best. *Electromagnetic Man: Health and Hazard in the Electrical Environment.* New York: St. Martin, 1989.

*29. Soyka, Fred. *The Ion Effect: How Air Electricity Rules Your Life and Health.* New York: Dutton, 1977.

30. Various Chinese Experts and the Staff of the People's Medical Publishing House of Beijing, China. *The

*Chinese Way to a Long and Healthy Life.* New York: Bell Publishing Co., 1984.

31.   Willis, Isaac M.D. "Discoid Lupus Erythematosus." Paper from Lupus Foundation of America Greater Arizona Chapter, Inc., Phoenix, AZ.

BIBLIOGRAPHY

# INDEX

## Index of Sources

True science seeks the possibility of the preconceived impossible by exploring the simple within the complex and the complex within the simple that the possibilities of those impossibilities may be known.